Leilson Bezerra
Ricardo Edvan
Marcos Araújo

# Transition Period in Cows: Nutrition, Metabolism and Metabolic Disease

AF153076

Leilson Bezerra
Ricardo Edvan
Marcos Araújo

# Transition Period in Cows: Nutrition, Metabolism and Metabolic Disease

**LAP LAMBERT** Academic Publishing

**Impressum / Imprint**

Bibliografische Information der Deutschen Nationalbibliothek: Die Deutsche Nationalbibliothek verzeichnet diese Publikation in der Deutschen Nationalbibliografie; detaillierte bibliografische Daten sind im Internet über http://dnb.d-nb.de abrufbar.
Alle in diesem Buch genannten Marken und Produktnamen unterliegen warenzeichen-, marken- oder patentrechtlichem Schutz bzw. sind Warenzeichen oder eingetragene Warenzeichen der jeweiligen Inhaber. Die Wiedergabe von Marken, Produktnamen, Gebrauchsnamen, Handelsnamen, Warenbezeichnungen u.s.w. in diesem Werk berechtigt auch ohne besondere Kennzeichnung nicht zu der Annahme, dass solche Namen im Sinne der Warenzeichen- und Markenschutzgesetzgebung als frei zu betrachten wären und daher von jedermann benutzt werden dürften.

Bibliographic information published by the Deutsche Nationalbibliothek: The Deutsche Nationalbibliothek lists this publication in the Deutsche Nationalbibliografie; detailed bibliographic data are available in the Internet at http://dnb.d-nb.de.
Any brand names and product names mentioned in this book are subject to trademark, brand or patent protection and are trademarks or registered trademarks of their respective holders. The use of brand names, product names, common names, trade names, product descriptions etc. even without a particular marking in this works is in no way to be construed to mean that such names may be regarded as unrestricted in respect of trademark and brand protection legislation and could thus be used by anyone.

Coverbild / Cover image: www.ingimage.com

Verlag / Publisher:
LAP LAMBERT Academic Publishing
ist ein Imprint der / is a trademark of
OmniScriptum GmbH & Co. KG
Heinrich-Böcking-Str. 6-8, 66121 Saarbrücken, Deutschland / Germany
Email: info@lap-publishing.com

Herstellung: siehe letzte Seite /
Printed at: see last page
**ISBN: 978-3-659-58511-1**

Zugl. / Approved by: Bom Jesus city, Piauí State, Brazil, Federal University of Piauí, 2014

## Dedication

This book is dedicated first to God, the Great Architect of the Universe, who gave me life and allowed his creation to be possible.

Also dedicated to my beloved wife, Karla nayalle, my son and my parents John Petter Francisco Bezerra and Maria Perpetua, and my sister Maria Augusta for the confidence and all the dedicated love.

And finally, to my teachers, professors and colleagues who share my knowledge and learning.

# Table of contents

# 1. Introduction

The success of the production cycle of a cow is determined by its production level, the postpartum recovery reproductive function and absence of pathology. Undoubtedly, the achievement of these objectives depends largely on the state of animal in its early days postpartum. So much so, that the level of production, the level of intake and blood parameters (NEFA, ketone bodies) in the first week postpartum are good indicators of the quality of initiating lactation (Grummer, Mashek, & Hayirli, 2004).

The energy balance is the result of the difference between the needs of the animal and food contributions. During last 2-4 weeks of gestation there is an increase substantial energy requirements due to fetal development and the needs of colostrum synthesis. This is accompanied by a decrease in the ingestion of materials dry. These two circumstances are often responsible for the development of a negative energy balance that initiates A few weeks before delivery. Cattle have the ability to compensate for deficits food energy through the mobilization of body fat. However, an excess mobilization of fat leads to disease and reproductive problems

The metabolic diseases or disorders of production are caused by an imbalance of nutrients that enter the animal organism (glicídeos, proteins, minerals, and water), your metabolism and graduates through feces, urine, milk and fetus. Nutritional imbalances affecting livestock are produced because the supply or use of foods is not meet nutritional requirements for maintenance, growth, production, reproduction (Martinez et al., 2014). When these imbalances are of short duration and are not too severe, the metabolism of the animal can compensate by using their body reserves. However, if the imbalance is severe or moderate but persistent animal body depletes its reserves and disease occurs (Wittwer, 2000). Unfortunately, most of these diseases has an effect difficult to perceive and act by limiting the production of the species of a persistently causing a decrease in the profitability of livestock enterprise.

The transition period consists of two phases, the first being formed by last three weeks before calving and the second by the first three weeks postpartum. This period is marked by changes, some of these are related to Alterations Increases in energy requirements driven by both fetal needs and lactogenesis, endocrine and metabolic preparing cows for childbirth and lactation (Morgante et al., 2012; Piccione et al., 2012).

According to most recent National Animal Health Monitoring System for dairy cattle (National Animal Health Monitoring System, 2008), leading causes of morbidity in dairy cattle are clinical mastitis, lameness, infertility, retained placenta, milk fever, reproductive problems, and displaced abomasum. Of cows removed from herds, about 53% leave for one or more of the above reasons. Additionally, the rate of mortality of cows in U.S. dairy herds is nearly 6%, with 43% of these related to periparturient health issues, and likely a large portion of those classified as ñunknownò (25%) occurring as a result of complications from the above. Overall, 16.2% of the cows that are permanently removed from a dairy herd are removed before 50 days in milk. These cows represent losses before the most profitable period of lactation. The relationship of the above disorders to excess prepartum body condition score (BCS) has been documented by numerous researchers and extensively reviewed (Bewley & Schultz, 2008). Briefly, cows with excessive body condition at calving, or excessive weight loss after calving, demonstrate overall decreased reproductive performance and increased likelihood of dystocia, retained placenta, metritis, milk fever, cystic ovaries, lameness, and mastitis as well as metabolic disorders, fatty liver, and ketosis.

## 2. Development

*2.1 The Importance of Transition Period*

An ancient Chinese curse states, in effect, ñMay you always live in interesting times.ò In this context, the transition period between late pregnancy and early lactation (also called the periparturient period) certainly is the most interesting stage of the lactation cycle. Although the length of time classified as the transition period has been defined differently by different authors, I define it as did Grummer (1995) as the last 3 wk before parturition to 3 wk after parturition. Most infectious diseases and metabolic disorders occur during this time. Milk fever, ketosis, retained fetal membranes, metritis, and displaced abomasum primarily impact cows during the periparturient period. Immunosuppression during the periparturient period (Mallard et al., 1988) leads to increased susceptibility to mastitis. Indeed, the incidence of environmental mastitis is greatest around parturition (Smith et al., 1985). Thus, the occurrence of health problems is centered disproportionately on this relatively short period, which certainly contributes to making this an ñinterestingò time for dairy producers. As stated by Goff and Horst (1997), ñThe transition from the pregnant, nonlactating state to the nonpregnant, lactating state is too often adisastrous experience for the cow. The well-being and profitability of the cow could be greatly enhanced by understanding those factors that account for the high disease incidence in periparturient cows.ò

Despite the prodigious output of research on the nutrition and physiology of transition cows, the transition period remains a problematic area on many dairy farms, and metabolic disorders continue to occur at economically important rates on commercial dairy farms (Burhans et al., 2003). Data recently summarized (Godden et al., 2003) indicate that approximately 25% of cows that left dairy herds in Minnesota from 1996 to 2001 did so during the first 60 DIM, with an uncertain additional

3

percentage leaving by the end of the lactation due in part to difficulty during the transition period. The economic ramifications of the loss of cows early in lactation together with the comprehensive costs associated with occurrence of the various metabolic disorders in both clinical and subclinical form are large. Therefore, research attention will continue to focus on understanding the biology of transition cows and implementing management schemes on dairy farms to optimize production and profitability on these farms (Overton and Waldron, 2004). The success of the transition period effectively determines the profitability of the cow during that lactation. Nutritional or management limitations during this time may impede the ability of the cow to reach maximal milk production. The primary challenge faced by cows is a sudden and marked increase of nutrient requirements for milk production, at a time when DMI, and thus nutrient supply, lags far behind. This situation is exhibited clearly in data presented by Bell (11), which have been plotted in Figure 1.

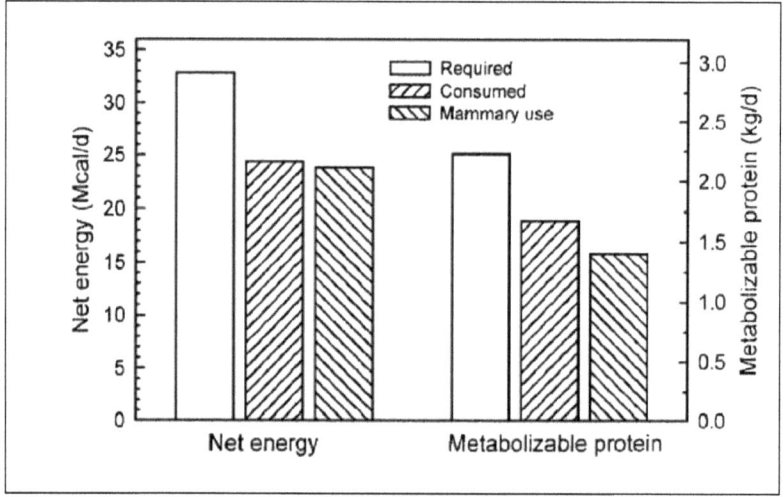

Figure 1. Calculations of amounts of NEL and metabolizable protein required, consumed, and utilized by lactating mammary gland of healthy dairy cows at 4 d postpartum. (Adapted from Bell, 1992).

*2.2 Biology and Phisiology of Dairy Cows During the Transition Period*

Transition cow biology and management has become a focal point for research in nutrition and physiology during the past 15 yr. First, it was recognized that many of the metabolic disorders afflicting cows during the periparturient period are interrelated in their occurrence and are related to the diet fed during the prepartum period (Curtis et al., 1985). They determined that increased energy content of the diet fed during the prepartum period was associated with decreased incidence of displaced abomasum and that increased protein content of this diet was associated with decreased incidences of retained placenta and ketosis (Curtis et al., 1985). Although the strategy for prevention of milk fever was to feed a prepartum diet low in Ca at that time, Ca content of the prepartum diet was not related to the occurrence of milk fever in their study. These results led to substantial investigation of the biological relationships underpinning these epidemiological relationships.

The biology of dairy cow health and reproductive performance is multifactorial and complex. High producing dairy cows have been described as ñmetabolic athletesà. However, 30 to 50% of dairy cows are affected by some form of metabolic or infectious disease around the time of calving. Dairy cattle have been selected to re-partition nutrients in support of milk production, a process described as homeorhesis (Bauman, 2000) in which homeostatic mechanisms are at least partially and temporarily overridden, including a period of physiologic insulin resistance. Essentially all peripartum dairy cattle experience: a period of insulin resistance, reduced feed intake, negative energy balance, lipolysis, and weight loss in early lactation; hypocalcemia in the days after calving; reduced immune function for 1 to 2 weeks before, and 2 to 3 weeks after calving; and, bacterial contamination of the uterus for 2 to 3 weeks after calving.

The body needs glucose for at least the following five components: nervous system, fat, muscle, fetuses and mammary gland. The increase of the bodies ketone also occur by ingestion of food ketogenic (amended silage rich in butyric acid oilseed cakes still very rich in fats and also feed unbalanced (excess albumin and failure of fiber). When ketosis is produced by these aforementioned problems without the participation of other disease is referred to as Primary ketosis. But it is not uncommon ketosis occur as a result of other diseases (Puerperal disorders, mastitis, hepatitis, or other traumatic reticuloperitonite indigestion) which causes changes in metabolism of carbohydrates or the inappetence, determining insufficient food intake; then we speak of ketosis secondary (Heidrich et al., 1980).

These factors, as well as dramatic changes in circulating progesterone, estrogen, and cortisol concentrations contribute to asubstantial reduction of immune function, in particular of neutronphils, at this time (Kehrli et al., 1989; Goff and Horst, 1997). Specifically, innate immunity from neutrophils is a primary means of immune response in the uterus and neutrophil migration and phagocytic and oxidative activity are associated with the risk of retained placenta (RP) (Kimura et al., 2002), metritis, and endometritis (Hammon et al., 2006). Yet, while metabolic (e.g. ketosis and fatty liver) and uterine disease are excessively common, only a minority of cows experience these problems, between herds or even within a herd in which cows apparently have similar nutritional and management experiences. Prediction or early detection of which cows

have health problems is an important goal. Interestingly, although most dairy cattle do not have the issues of obesity that preoccupy human health research, peripartum cattle do go through a period of substantial insulin resistance that has elements in common with Type 2 diabetes (Lucy, 2004), with the important difference that cows have low blood glucose. Dairy cattle also go through a period of

6

substantial lipolysis and a high flux of fatty acids to the liver. High circulating non-esterified fatty acid (NEFA) concentrations are a major risk factor for fatty liver and may also have direct effects on neutrophil function (Scalia et al., 2006). Because of both high metabolic demands and pathogen challenges, cattle also routinely experience substantial oxidative stress at the same time (Sordillo and Aitken, 2009).

To achieve the economic objective of pregnancy within 80 to 120 days after the previous calving, the uterus must return to a condition to support a new pregnancy, and a regular estrus cycle mustbe re-established. This is the result of a complex set of interactions and endocrine signalling among the brain, liver, ovaries and uterus. While a few research groups have begun to look at the links between energy metabolism and reproductive function, there is a gap in examining the large intervening component of uterine dis ease, which is at play in as many as half of all cows. Uterine health problems (RP, metritis (uterine infection causing systemic illness in early lactation), and endometritis (chronic low-grade uterine infection and inflammation between 3 and 9 weeks postpartum) affect up to half of dairy cows in the first 60 days postpartum (Sheldon et al., 2006).

The ultimate metabolic impact of the conceptus on its dam is best represented in terms of the nutrient requirements of the whole gravid uterus (i.e., uterine tissues, placenta, fetal membranes and fetus).

To Fetal Metabolisrn, during late pregnancy, fetal metabolic rate, represented as weight-specific oxygen consumption, is approximately twice that of the dam (Reynolds et al., 1986). Most of the carbon and nitrogen required for fetal growth and metabolism is supplied by glucose (directly and via its fetal-placental intermediate, lactate) and amino acids. This is clearly evident in Table 1, in which metabolic balance sheets for specific nutrient contributions to energy and nitrogen requirements in the late-gestation bovine fetus are presented.

Table 1. Fetal sources and requirements of energy and nitrogen in late-pregnant cows[a]

| Nutriente | Energy (kca/day) | Nitrogen (g/Day) |
|---|---|---|
| Sources | | |
| Glucose and Lactate[bcd] | 775 | - |
| Amino acids[d] | 1,306 | 38 |
| Acetateb | 255 | - |
| Total | 2,336 | 38 |
| Requirements | | |
| Tissue deposition[e] | 605 | 12 |
| Heat[bd] | 1,605 | - |
| Urea[d] | 125 | 23 |
| Total | 2,335 | 35 |

[a]Data from different breeds are scaled to a fetal weight of 35 kg at 250 d of pregnancy to represent the Holstein breed (Bell et al., 1992).
[b]Comline and Silver (1976).
[c]Reynolds et al. (1986).
[d]Ferrell (1991).
[e]Bell et al. (1992).

The debit and credit sides of the metabolic ledger balance surprisingly well, despite considerable uncertainty about some of the estimates. Direct measurement of fetal oxidation of glucose and lactate indicates that in well-fed ewes these substrates account for no more than 50 to 60% of fetal respiration (Hay et al., 1983). Placental transport of short- and long-chain fatty acids and ketones is limited in ruminants (Bell, 1993). Fetal uptake of maternal acetate was estimatedt o contribute, at most, 10 to 15% of fetal respiratory fuel in late-pregnant cows (Comline and Silver, 1976).

The remaining 30 to 40% of substrate for oxidation seems to be amino acids, which, based on measurements of fetal urea production, are extensively catabolized by the wellnourished fetus (Faichney and White, 1987). This would seem to be an unusual metabolic situation in a rapidly growing organism. However, it is consistent with observations that fetal protein deposition accounts for, at most, 50% of the fetal net uptake of amino acids in sheep (Lemons et al., 1976; Meier et al.,

1981) and cattle (Reynolds et al., 1986; Ferrell, 1991). In fact, the data summarized in Table 1 suggest that only 32% of amino acid nitrogen taken up by the late-gestation bovine fetus is deposited in tissue protein. This means that the fetal requirement for metabolizable amino acids is approximately three times the net requirement for fetal growth. For example, we recently reported an average rate of crude protein deposition of 74 gld in Holstein fetuses between d 190 and 270 of gestation, with a projected mean birth weight of 45 kg (Bell et al., 1992). From this, the metabolizable amino acid requirement for fetal growth was estimated to be about 220 gld. In contrast, the nutrient requiremenfto r fat deposition in fetal ruminants is relatively insignificant. In our Holstein cow study, the average rate of fetal fat deposition during late pregnancy was a mere 12 g/dl (Bell et al., 1992), accounting for less than 5% of theestimated fetal energy requirement (Table 1). This is consistent with the low body fat content (< 30 glkg) of newborn calves (Ellenberger et al., 1950). In sheep, which are similarly lean at birth, the modest rate of fetal fat deposition has been attributed to placental impermeability to preformed long-chain fatty acids in the maternal circulation (Elphick et al., 1979) and a greatly reduced capacity for de novo fatty acid synthesis in fetala dipose tissue during latep regnancy (Vernon et al., 1981).

To Placental and Uterine Metabolism, the uteroplacental tissues (placentomes, endometrium, myometrium) account for less than 20% of the weight of the gravid uterus during late pregnancy. However, they consume 35 to 50% of oxygen and at least 65% of glucose taken up by the uterus in ewes (Meschia et al., 1980) and cows (Reynolds et al., 1986).

As previously discussed (Bell, 1993), most of this relatively intense metabolic activity must be confined to the placenta because most of the maternal and fetal blood perfusing the uteroplacental tissue mass is distributed to the placentomes. Although much of the glucose taken up by the uteroplacenta is undoubtedly oxidized to completion, a considerable fraction (30 to 40%) is converted

to lactate, which is released into maternal and fetal circulations (Meschia et al., 1980; Reynolds et al.,

1986).

Radiotracer studies have shown that the fetal portion is derived from metabolism of fetal glucose and

therefore represents recycling of fetal glucose carbon within the fetal-placental unit. In contrast,

lactate released into the maternal circulation is derived from caruncular and uterine tissue metabolism

of maternal glucose (Bassett, 1986). An additional, smaller fraction

of glucose taken up by the fetal placenta is metabolized to fructose and released back into the

umbilical circulation.

The high blood concentrations of this hexose in fetal ruminants is more a consequence of slow fetal

clearance and metabolism than of rapid placental production (Meznarich et al., 1987). Bovine

placental growth continues into late pregnancy, at least until approximately 230 d (Ferrell et al.,

1976). However, the rate of growth is modest, accounting for a net accretion of no more than about 7

g/d of CP. Greater rates of uteroplacental consumption of amino acids have been reported (Reynolds

et al., 1986; Ferrell, 1991), implying considerable placental catabolism. The nature of this process

remains uncertain in cattle, although some enzymatic capacity for placental ureagenesis has been

reported (Ferrell, 1988).

To summarize, the nonfetal components of the gravid uterus, especially the placenta, account for

large fractions of uterine oxygen and glucose consumption in cattle and sheep. In cows, but not in

ewes, the uteroplacental net consumption of amino acids is puzzlingly high. The gravid uterus also

takes up modest amounts of acetate and 3-hydroxybutyrate, metabolism of which is mostly confined

to the (presumably) maternal uteroplacental tissues (Bell, 1993; Bell, 1995).

## 2.3 Nutrition and Nutrient Requirements Transition Period

The period of transition between late pregnancy and early lactation presents an enormous metabolic challenge to the high-yielding dairy cow. Failure to adequately meet this challenge can result in a rangeo fearly postpartum health problems, some potentially fatal, and compromised lactation performance, as discussed elsewhere in this symposium (Grummer, 1995). Nutritional and other strategies to facilitate the periparturient transition should be based on a thorough understanding of the quality and quantityo of nutrients required to support conceptus growth during late pregnancy and milk synthesis during early lactation. The homeorhetic regulation of metabolic changes in nonuterine and nonmammary tissues, such as liver and adipose tissue, is also a vitally important consideration.

Energy is the main limiting nutrient in feed dairy cattle, as is required in much higher amount others. For some time the level of effect has been documented energy in the diet on reproductive performance of cows. In beef cows a diet with low energy pre and post calving interval causes more birth / first estrus, and lower birth rate. In dairy cows, this is due low intake of energy associated with a high production of milk, which causes a loss of weight and / or body condition after childbirth.

Requirements for NEL and metabolizable protein by healthy cows at 4 d postpartum exceeded intakes by 26 and 25%, respectively. Furthermore, calculated utilization of NEL and metabolizable protein by the mammary gland for milk production accounted for 97 and 83%, respectively, of intakes, leaving little to supply maintenance needs.

The constraints imposed by the deficient intakes, coupled with other stressors associated with parturition and adjustments to lactation; no doubt contribute to the high incidence of health disorders during the transition period. Survey data of disease incidence in transition cows vary widely, yet it is this variation itself that is perhaps so fascinating.

The recently calved cows have to give high yields. After birth, it is expected that milk bovine females reach peak production quickly and devise a new creates the first 85 days of lactation. This constitutes a formidable challenge. In addition, the ability of a cow to achieve this goal increases with adequate nutritional management during the transition from six weeks (Olson, 2002).

A series of physiological adaptations occur in dairy cows in early lactation, always aiming to milk production in detriment of other metabolic activities, such as the maintenance, growth and reproduction. These characteristics are related to changes in hormone serum concentrations favoring the supply of nutrients to the mammary gland to the detriment of other tissues (Matos, 1995) commonly called homeorrhesis (Bauman & Currie, 1980).

Soon after birth, the dry matter intake increases day after day until you reach the peak around the 10th. the 12th. week of lactation, while the peak milk yield is about 4 to 6 weeks postpartum (NRC, 1989). This difference in milk production and dry matter intake turn causes the experiment the animal during a period of ± 60 days negative nutritional imbalance (Santos et al. 1993), due to the mobilization of body reserves accumulated at the end lactation or dry period, some muscle or protein and calcium from the bones (Matos, 1995).

The primary goal of nutritional management strategies of dairy cows during the transition period should be to support the metabolic adaptations described above. Industry-standard nutritional management of dairy cows during the dry period consists of a 2-group nutritional scheme (Overton and Waldron, 2004). The NRC (2001) recommended that a diet containing approximately 1.25 Mcal/kg of NEL be fed from dry off until approximately 21 d before calving, and that a diet containing 1.54 to 1.62 Mcal/kg of NEL be fed during the last 3 wk preceding parturition. The primary rationale for feeding a lower energy diet during the early dry period is to minimize BCS gain during the dry period; furthermore, Dann et al. (2003) reported recently that supplying excessive energy to dairy cows during the early dry period may actually have detrimental carryover effects during the subsequent early lactation period. The nature of these carryover effects is not known.

One could speculate, however, that effects could be mediated through metabolic machinery responsible for tissue responsiveness to endocrine signals during the late prepartum period. In general, available information supports feeding the higher energy diet for two to three weeks prior to parturition (Corbett, 2002; Contreras et al., 2004). Results from 2 of these experiments indicated farm-specific negative effects on subsequent production and health if cows were fed the higher energy diet for the entire dry period (Contreras et al., 2004) or for an average of 37 d prepartum (Mashek and Beede, 2001). These responses may correspond to the negative carryover effects of overfeeding energy during the early dry period described by Dann et al. (2003). Furthermore, recent results (Contreras et al., 2004) support managing cows to achieve a BCS of approximately 3.0 at dry off rather than the traditional 3.5 to 3.75 BCSõ perhaps partially due to the decreased DMI associated with higherBCSduring the prepartum period (Hayirli et al., 2002). Studies conducted with limited replication indicate increased DMI and milk yield for cows of BCS 2 to 2.5 at calving versus those with a BCS of 3.5 to 4 on a 4-point scale (Garnsworthy and Topps, 1982a, 1982b; Treacher et al., 1986; Garnsworthy and Jones, 1987). These results are also consistent with those of Domecq et al. (1997), who reported that as BCS of cows at dry off increased, milk yield during the first 120 DIM decreased; furthermore, thinner cows that gained BCS during the dry period yielded more milk during the first 120 DIM. Collectively, results published in the scientific literature support the concept that cows of moderately lower BCS within a well-managed transition management system are more likely

13

to have positive transition period outcomes than cows of greater BCS due to their propensity to have increased DMI and potentially increased milk yield during early lactation.

Therefore, a calving should reserve around 10% of its weight in order to meet the common nutritional deficiency in early lactation.

The most critical phase in the life of the dairy cow lies in the first 21 days of lactation, where the strongest mobilization of fat and to a lesser extent body protein occurs mainly in the case of high-producing cows (Chilliard et al., 1983 ).

A cow 600 kg BW should have an additional 60 kg of body reserves. Each kg of body weight corresponds approximately 5 Mcal of net energy lactation and 320 grams of protein. Taking into account the needs of production of one kilogram of milk lie to 0.74 Mcal of net energy lactation and 90 grams of crude protein (CP), this cow has "reserve" the equivalent of 405 kg of milk (base power), ie (60 x 5/0, 74) and about 213 kg of milk based protein (60 x 320/90) (NRC, 1989). With that, the high producing cow has almost 2 times more energy reserves than protein reserves (Santos et al., 1993). The loss of live weight of the cow in early lactation is closely linked with individual capacity, since the animal mobilizes its body reserves to meet its production potential, resulting in considerable loss of weight

Use of supplemental fats and oils in diets for dairy cows has become a standard practice. Extensive researchhas been conducted to determine the effects of supplemental fats on milk yield and composition, intake, and digestion. A much smaller body of research is available concerning the effects of dietary fats on postabsorptive metabolism in dairy cows (Grummer, 1993; Palmquist, 1994).

These issues assume practical as well as academic importance; for example, concern often is expressed about whether dietary fat increases the likelihood of fatty liver development or decreased liver function. Dietary fat results in widespread metabolic changes in rodents, including increased peroxisomal and mitochondrial $b$-oxidation of FA (Kumamoto and Ide, 1998; Malewiak et al., 1988), decreased esterification of FA (Malewiak et al., 1988), altered profiles and clearance of plasma lipoproteins (Lambert et al., 1998), induction of xenobiotic metabolizing enzymes (Yang et al., 1993), and altered responsiveness to hormonal signals (Dax et al., 1990). Parallel changes in dairy cows could be important adaptations to use of dietary fat. Furthermore, because many of these changes in lipid metabolism induced by dietary fat also occur during starvation or negative energy balance in rodents, they might also be important adaptations during the transition period in dairy cows. It has been proposed that dietary fat may help to decrease concentrations of NEFA and help to prevent occurrence of ketosis (Kronfeld, 1982). Dietary long-chain fatty acids are absorbed into the lymphatic system and do not pass first through the liver. This fat can provide energy for peripheral tissues and the mammary gland. Kronfeld's hypothesis is that the increased energy availability would in turn decrease mobilization of body fat and decrease NEFA concentrations.

Despite available information (Skaar et al., 1989; Grum et al., 1996; Burhans and Bell, 1998; Douglas et al., 1998; Bertics and Grummer, 1999), indicating that added fat fed to cows during the prepartum period does not decrease plasma NEFA concentrations, advancement of this hypothesis by various commercial interests in the dairy industry has continued. Grum et al. (1996) determined that feeding fat (6.7% of diet DM) to cows during the entire dry period virtually abolished accumulation of triglycerides in liver during the immediate peripartal period; however, cows fed fat also had decreased DMI during the dry period. A subsequent experiment (Douglas et al., 1998) determined

15

that the reduction in liver triglycerides was mostly attributable to the decreased DMI of cows fed added fat during the dry period. As indicated above, Doepel et al. (2002) reported that cows fed high-energy diets during the prepartum period had decreased peripartal concentrations of NEFA in plasma and tended to have decreased postpartum liver triglyceride concentrations. The increase in energy content of the prepartum diet was achieved by a combination of increasing NFC content as reported above and addition of tallow at 2.2% of DM. The preponderance of results reported above suggest that the results of Doepel et al. (2002) occurred as a consequence of changes made in the NFC content of the diet rather than in the fat content of the diet. Anecdotal reports from some practitioners in the dairy industry have indicated beneficial effects of administering dietary fat by oral drench to cows during the immediate postpartum period, and dietary fat sources are commonly included in commercially available mixtures administered orally to fresh cows. Pickett et al. (2003b) administered 454 g/d of a commercially available fat supplement (82% fatty acids by weight) by oral drench for the first 3 d of lactation; administration of fat did not affect concentrations of NEFA and BHBA in plasma and triglycerides in liver during the postpartum period, and tended to decrease DMI and milk yield during the first 21 d of lactation.

Significant progress in understanding the metabolic adaptations that dairy cows make as they transition from a nonlactating to lactating state has enabled continual development of specific nutritional strategies to support these metabolic adaptations (Overton and Waldron, 2004). Overall, research supports 2-group nutritional management schemes for dry cows to minimize overfeeding during the early dry period and to increase energy supply to dairy cows during the late prepartum period. Although confirming studies are required, recent evidence suggests that metabolism and performance of transition cows is more sensitive to total energy supplied by carbohydrate than the form of that carbohydrate (i.e., starch versus highly digestible NDF). Efforts to improve the energy status of dairy cows during the periparturient period and decrease NEFA release from adipose tissue by feeding added dietary fat sources or trans-10, cis-12 CLA have not resulted in improved metabolism or consistently improved performance (Overton and Waldron, 2004). Although the dogma has been that there is little potential to nutritionally affect hepatic metabolism of NEFA extracted from the circulation, recent evidence suggests that nutrients such as choline and essential fatty acids may increase rates of hepatic export of NEFA as triglycerides in VLDL (Overton and Waldron, 2004). Calcium mobilization in support of lactation can be facilitated effectively by lowering the DCAD of the diet fed during the prepartum period; however, the degree to which the DCAD must be lowered to sufficiently alleviate hypocalcemia remains controversial. Our understanding of periparturient nutritional physiology continues to evolve; however, the substantial variation in response to nutritional manipulation that occurs on commercial dairy farms is a reminder that transition cow management is a multifaceted issue.

In the case of medium and high animal production is essential the supply of fodder quality associated with supplementation concentrated. To increase efficiency reproduction of dairy cows is essential to maximize consumption food especially in early lactation. Improving energy balance by increasing energy intake (for example use of protected fat) in the diet reduces days first and improves ovulation postpartum design. The content of fat diet may need to spend 4% of the diet DM in the early postpartum period. Cottonseed appears to be the most economical method today for supplemental fat in diets of dairy cows when available in the region.

The supply of protein is more easily solved through the use of legumes and / or protein supplements, including sources of non-protein nitrogen (urea, ammonia). Should avoid the use of high levels of

17

protein, especially degradable protein. Using protein sources containing acids mono-and polyunsaturated fatty long chain as flour fish has been shown to increase the milk production and performance reproductive health of dairy cows (Canfield et al., 1990).

Our understanding of the biology of transition cows is in its infancy relative to the knowledge base of cows at peak lactation or beyond. Research attention to this critical area has virtually exploded in the last few years and substantial progress is likely during the next decade. Some areas in which increased understanding is critical include 1) the control of DMI during the periparturient period, 2) quantification of nutrient supply during this period when DMI and gut capacity are changing rapidly, 3) interactions among nutrition, metabolism, and the immune system, 4) metabolic regulation in, and interactions among, liver, adipose tissue, muscle, and the digestive tract in support of the initiation of lactation, and 5) effects of body condition on

transition success and metabolic responses to different transition management strategies (Drackley, 1999).

*2.4 Negative Energy Balance (NEB)*

The negative energy balance (NEB) is a physiological period for which all the cow passes. But this can be reduced and its effects can be reduced and cause less alterations in the milk production of cows and breeding. For this an appropriate nutritional management should be performed. Most important to reverse the NEB is the availability of food: palatable, easy access, good quality and quantity. Thus ensuring maximum dry matter intake (Butler, 2004).

During the periparturient period, high yielding dairy cows experience major changes in energy metabolism (Bauman, 2000). With the onset of lactation, the added metabolic activities of the mammary gland increase the total energy requirements by approximately fourfold. A pronounced energy deficit develops because voluntary feed intake is insufficient to meet this increased energy expenditure, and is met by mobilizing lipids from white adipose tissue (WAT) (Bauman & Currie 1980, Bell 1995, Barber et al. 1997, Bauman 2000).

Despite this shortfall, partitioning of nutrients to the mammary gland is favored, and represents over 70% of available energy (ingested and endogenous).The metabolic context of the nutritional insufficiency of early lactation is, however, different from that associated with fasting or undernutrition. First, increased demand, not decreased provision of nutrients, is the primary cause of the undernourished state in early lactation. Second, because the undernutrition associated with the onset of milk synthesis confers no direct benefits to the mother, lactation must call on additional hormonal and cellular adaptations to harness maternal energy metabolism (Bauman & Currie 1980, Bell 1995, Vernon & Pond 1997, Bauman 2000).

One to two weeks before calving, food intake decreases, leading to NEB. NEB becomes more pronounced two to three postpartum due to increased nutrient demands in early lactation weeks. The first 60 days postpartum cows increases milk production. The early lactation leads to a huge demand of nutrients especially in high producing dairy cows. These do not have a compensatory consumption of food because they can not consume the necessary. When they go through a period of NEB increases the levels of non-esterified fatty acids (NEFA) in the blood stream, along with a fall in blood glucose levels, insulin and insulin-like growth factor (IGF-1) factor. These metabolic changes lead to a decrease in pulse LH (luteinizing hormone), needed to stimulate the development of ovarian follicles and also reducing the ovarian response to gonadotropins. The delay or low steroid production in the ovaries, estrogen and progesterone in follicles after ovulation, promotes delayed uterine involution and the restoration of their functions (Santos, 2005, Butler 2004).

The severity and duration of negative energy balance are more strongly related to dry matter intake (r = 0.73) than for milk production (r = -0.25) (Villa-Godoy et al. 1988) and this in turn with the animal's body condition at calving (Butler, 2000).

Parallel to this whole box of dry matter intake and milk production (energy balance), we follicle growth, ovulation, fertilization and embryonic development, these factors closely related. According to Butler (2000) the intensity of negative energy balance in the 3 to 4 weeks postpartum is highly correlated with days to first ovulation. NEB entails mobilization of body fat. The amount of fatty acids that can be metabolized by the liver is low. When this process the fatty acids entering the liver is saturated, are transformed into triglycerides that accumulate in hepatocytes, featuring a picture of steatosis or "fatty liver", further aggravating the process. Acetyl-CoA would be incorporated into the tricarboxylic acid cycle is then used for the synthesis of acetoacetate, β-hydroxybutyrate) and acetone, these substances are also known β-hydroxybutyrate (as ketone bodies, when present in increased concentrations in the blood, cause the clinical condition known as ketosis (Souza, 2003).

Accumulation of the β-hydroxybutyrate in transition period, concentrations of NEFA and triglycerides in the liver were higher in cows in which the first dominant follicle postpartum not ovulated, compared with those presented β-hydroxybutyrate ovulatory follicles. The strong negative relationship between NEFA concentrations and ovulatory status with the FD shows that higher circulating levels may act by inhibiting the production of follicular estradiol and ovulation. The sites are potential inhibition in the hypothalamus, in the frequency of LH pulses, and the sensitivity of follicles to metabolic stimuli such as insulin and IGF-1 (Butler, 2004).

BEN generates losses in body condition of cows, leading to anovulation and prolonged postpartum anestrus, lengthens the period from calving to first service and reduces fertility. Malnutrition also inhibits estrous behavior of cows due to lower estrogen response of the central nervous system as drop in the number of receptors in the CNS occurs. It is possible that endocrine and metabolic factors associated with NEB occurring during the growth of follicles in early stages of growth will eventually affect the quality of oocytes and CL (corpus luteum) subsequent to ovulation already in the period of insemination. Preantral follicles destined to ovulate weeks later, may have changed their quality due to metabolic factors during development (Santos, 2005).

The effect of undernutrition on reproduction are often viewed as a pathological condition which is caused by any defects in the reproductive system originated from nutritional deficiency. Although anovulation proper nutrition postpartum cows is undesirable, the inhibition of reproduction during periods of reduced availability energy is a common phenomenon in most mammals, and is probably reflects the activation mechanisms Physiological that reduce the likelihood of ovulation during periods of inadequate supply of energy. the mechanisms by which changes the energy balance affect reproductive function are not direct consequences of inadequate supply of nutrients but occur due to action metabolic signals that regulate ovarian function and hipofisiária.Cows that cycled later and anestrus presented progressive NEB mainly acyclic. In experiment (Thatcher, 2005) found that the dietary intake of cows in anestrus was continuously lower than cows that cycled. Apart from ingesting less in the first week postpartum, as time went on the difference between the intake of cows in anestrus increased more and more.

Britt (1994) placed as hypothesized that the effects of negative energy balance in reproduction of dairy cows is not only associated with period necessary to first postpartum ovulation but also with oocyte viability of the ovulatory follicle and the body CL ovulation that results from the follicle. According to this author, the time period for which a primary follicle develops into a ovulatory follicle may be 80-100 days. This is important evidence that metabolic factors may influence the rapid follicle development. It is conceivable that changes in metabolism occurred during periods of energy balance negative, can influence the follicles destined for ovulation the later, during the period of estrus. Following this line of thought Kendrick et al. (1997) marked at random cows 20 milk to receive two separate treatments with consumption High energy content (3.6%) and low (3.2%) of their body weight. the Follicles were aspirated transvaginally twice a week, and the oocytes were classified according to their density the cumulus and ooplasm homogeneity. Cows in better balance energy (high energy), had higher levels of IGF-I intrafollicular and progesterone in plasma, and also tended to produce more oocytes classified as good.

The return quickly to the estrous cycle, it is important to that conception occurs more rapidly. The time required for the first ovulation determines and limits the number of estrus cycles that may occur before the beginning of insemination. Typically, are present in flocks where less than 15% cows entering the estrus does not occur until 50 days after delivery. The expression of estrus and conception increase every cycle estrus after the third postpartum estrus.

For transition period is the shortest possible and that the reproductive performance of dairy cow is high is necessary to maximize the intake of dry matter (DM) and minimize the amount of negative energy balance during the early lactation. Efforts to minimize the nutritional extent and duration of negative energy balance can improve reproductive performance. The first and most important factor that affects energy intake in dairy cows is the availability food (Grant and Albright, 1995). Therefore, it can be concluded that cows milk must at all times be palatable diet high quality available to ensure maximum dry matter intake (IMS). However, IMS is limited during late gestation and early lactation (Santos, 1996), which may compromise the total intake of energy and reproductive performance. Many managements strategies Nutrition has been proposed to increase energy intake during early lactation. Food with high forage quality, increase in concentrate ratio: bulky, or addition of fat supplementation in diets are some of the many ways to increase energy intake in cows.

There is also a compromise on embryo survival. It is important that an early return to cyclicity with a view to an early design. The moment of the first ovulation determines and after delivery limits the number of estrus cycle occurring before the beginning of insemination. Generally in most dairy herds, less than 20% of cows should be anovulatory 60 days postpartum. The expression of estrus, conception rate and embryo survival improved when cows were cycling before an estrus synchronization program for the first postpartum insemination (Santos et al., 2004b) . Butler (2004) and quoting Lucy and Crooker, 2001 also reported there is a positive relationship between conception rate and early onset of ovulatory cycles postpartum. Conception rate increases over the course of the cycles, probably due to the improvement in progesterone profiles.

NEB is a physiological period for which all the cow passes. But this can be reduced and its effects can be reduced and cause less alterations in the milk production of cows and breeding. For this an appropriate nutritional management should be performed. According to Santos and Sá Filho (2006), the most important to reverse the BEN is the availability of food: palatable, easy access, good quality and quantity. Thus ensuring maximum dry matter intake. Besides the nutritional management should also pay attention to the reproductive and health management during the transition period. Thus the cow can reverse endocrine and metabolic changes mentioned can return to reproductive activities.

In the sequel will be reported major diseases or metabolic disorders affecting cows in der transition period.

*2.5Major Metabolic Diseases: Ketosis and Fatty Liver Syndrome*

Ketosis and Fatty Liver Syndrom is a metabolic disorder which often goes undiagnosed and leads to constricted performance and an impairment of general condition. It´s primarily occurs 2-7 weeks after calving (Gillund, Reksen, Grohn, & Karlberg, 2001) and occurs in consequence of negative energy balance, which will promote fat ana mobilização form of triacylglycerides (TGL). Before reaching the liver, TGL lose ester molecule in order to facilitate the conduction blood. Upon arriving at the liver TGL will be transformed into ketone bodies ketone bodies, acetoacetate (AcAc) and acetone (Ac) can be reduced to β-hydroxybutyrate (BHB) in an enzymatic reaction or decarboxylated to generate energy (Nielsen & Ingvartsen, 2004).

In early lactation, dairy cows high-yielding production suffer a variety of metabolic changes derived from energy deficiency, due to poor dry matter ingestion and high milk production, which are factors that predispose to ketosis (Chapinal et al., 2011) . A study to describe the prevalence of primary subclinical ketosis in New Zealand demonstrated age and calving interval are predisposing factors to the onset of ketosis (Compton, McDougall, Young & Bryan, 2014). Already Fatty Liver represents the major factor predisposing body condition score because fat and very fat cows have to have the disorder in the postpartum period. Furthermore, the Fatty liver may be a secondary complication to the cow to have a negative energy balance. Once developed fatty liver, and due to the low rate of export triglyceride in the form of lipoproteins, fatty liver persist for a long period. Reduction of fatty deposits in the liver is usually initiated when the cow enters positive energy balance, and end exhausted in the course of several weeks (Chapinal et al., 2012).

In the period between the end of late gestation and early lactation, there is a marked change from the dry matter intake by females. In cows reduction in consumption in this period is even more pronounced than for the heifers as shown in Figure 2. Over the first 30 days postpartum, when there is the peak of lactation, also observed consumption capacity suboptimal mobilization of body reserves for milk production, and often weight loss. The observed negative energy balance is due to insufficient nutrients necessary for lactation by dietary intake, because at this stage there is a priority of nutrients by the mammary gland (Leroy, Vanholde, Van Knegsel, Garcia-Ispierto & Bols, 2008) mediated by limiting the consumption capacity, causing a serious change in blood metabolites and hematological profile of animals (Piccione et al., 2012; Bezerra et al., 2013). With the advance of lactation (60 days postpartum), known as an intermediary period, milk production begins to decrease in the order of 2.5 % per week, while the voluntary intake increases gradually. Finally, at 90 days post partum, post- peak DM intake milk production continues to decrease gradually (NRC, 2008).

These responses, exaggerated by moderate under nutrition status in pregnant animals, are mediated by reduced tissue sensitivity and responsiveness to insulin, associated with decreased tissue expression of the insulin-responsive facilitative glucose transporter (GLUT4) (Bell & Bauman 1997). Peripheal tissue responses to insulin remain severely attenuated during early lactation but recover as the animal progresses through mid-lactation (Guesnet, Massoud & Demarne 1991, Bell & Bauman 1997, Sasaki 2002).

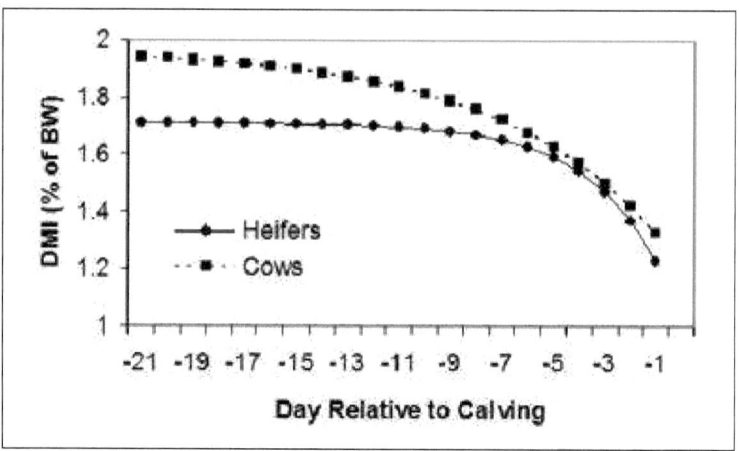

Figure 2. Dry matter intake comparative between cows and heifers during the transition period (Grummer, Mashek & Hayirli, 2004)

Thus, during the period of NEB, key hormone expression and tissue responsiveness alter to increase lipolysis and decrease lipogenesis, causing high levels of non-esterified fatty acids (NEFA) and б-hydroxybutyrate (BHB) concentration which are indicative of lipid mobilization and fatty acid oxidation (Sakha, Ameri & Rohbakhsh, 2006, Wathes et al., 2009). Excessive fat mobilization can induce an imbalance in he patic carbohydrate and fat metabolism, which may result in ketosis (Goff & Horst, 1997).

Fatty liver occurs when blood levels are elevated NEFA. This is dramatically raising birth. The liver's ability to grasp the NEFA is proportional to their concentration in the blood. The NEFA taken up by the liver are esterified to triglycerides or oxidized in mitochondria or peroxisomes (microsomes). TGL can be stored or exported as part of a low density lipoprotein. Compared with other species, the export capacity of liver triglycerides in ruminants is low, not knowing the cause. Under circumstances where an increase is produced in the liver uptake of NEFA (for example, when there are low levels of glucose and insulin in the blood), the esterification of fatty acids and accumulation of triglycerides in the liver occurs (Andresen, 2001). Complete oxidation of NEFA forms $CO_2$. Incomplete oxidation produces ketone bodies (especially acetoacetate and beta- hydroxy - butyrate. Formation of ketone bodies is also favored when blood levels of glucose and insulin are low, partly due to increased mobilization of fatty acids from tissue adipose. Low levels of insulin may increase the oxidation of fatty acids by reduction in malonyl -CoA concentration in hepatocytes and reduced sensitivity of the -1 carnitine palmitoiltrasferasa action of malonyl -CoA. Carnitine palmitoyltransferase - 1 is responsible for the translocation of fatty acids from the cytosol to the mitochondria for oxidation; action is inhibited by malonyl - CoA. Propionic acid is anti - ketogenic, probably due to its indirect effects in promoting insulin secretion and its direct effects on hepatic metabolism.

In the case of Fatty Liver Syndrome the deposition of TAG in liver is the consequence of mobilization of NEFA from adipose tissue exceeding capabilities of liver for oxidation and secretion of lipids (Gross, Schwarz, Eder, Van Dorland & Bruckmaier, 2013). Cows with fatty liver have greater adipose stores and mobilize more TAG, which leads to greater plasma NEFA concentrations, because adipose tissue from cows with fatty liver is less responsive to lipogenic substances and more responsive to lipolytic substances. Furthermore, cows with fatty liver have decreased fatty acid oxidation, hepatic apolipoprotein synthesis and lipid secretion, as indicated by decreased plasma apolipoprotein and lipid concentrations and decreased serum lecithin: cholesterol acyltransferase (LCAT) activity (Bobe, Young & Beitz, 2004). Besides disturbances in lipid metabolism, cows with fatty liver also have disturbances in glucose metabolism: Cows with fatty liver are either hyperinsulinemic-hyperglycemic or hypoinsulinemic-hypoglycemic (Holtenius, 1991), because either peripheral glucose uptake is decreased, indicating insulin resistance, or insulin and glucagon secretion and, therefore, hepatic gluconeogenesis are decreased. Furthermore, plasma amino acids are decreased. In summary, the availability of glucose, amino acids, and lipids for peripheral tissues is decreased in cows with fatty liver.

The diagnosis is made by clinical history, clinical signs and laboratory tests. The confirmation must be made by measurement of serum blood glucose (<50 mg/100 ml) b-hydroxybutyrate (> 14.4 mg / dl). The presence of ketones in the urine ("Ketostick") also assists in confirmation. The subclinical ketosis is characterized by a б-hydroxybutyrate (BHB) concentration in blood serum and milk (Figure 3; Herdt, Dart & Neuder, 2001). To generate this metabolic situation, an animal model was created. The model, based on group-specific interaction of dietary energy supply and body condition, is appropriate for testing the medical effectiveness of treating this kind of ketosis and its concomitants (Denis-Robichaud, Dubuc, Lefebvre & DesCôteaux, 2014; Campos, González, Coldebella & Lacerda, 2005). Research has been tested other forms of diagnosis as a magnetic resonance-based metabolomics. Sun et al. (2014) observed that plasma [1]H-nuclear magnetic resonance-based metabolomics, coupled with pattern recognition analytical methods, not only has the sensitivity and specificity to distinguish cows with clinical and subclinical ketosis from healthy controls, but also has the potential to be developed into a clinically useful diagnostic tool that could contribute to a further understanding of the disease mechanisms.

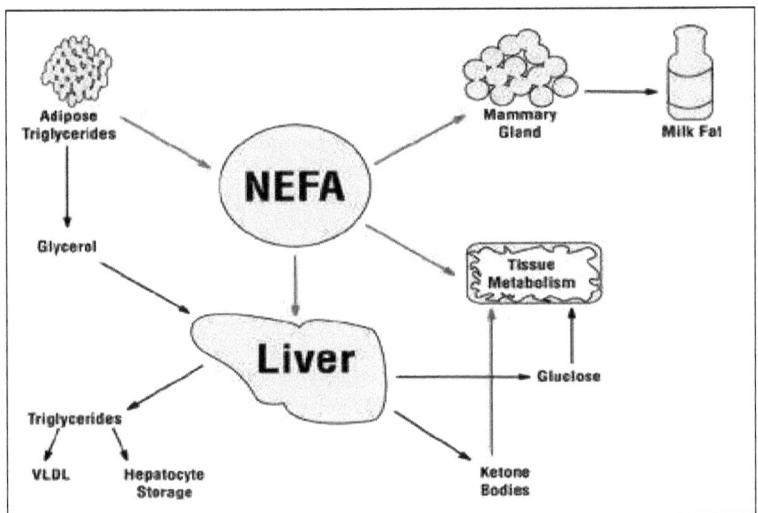

Figure 3: Non-esterfied fatty acids can be used as a sensitive indicator of energy balance in blood and milk. (Herdt, Dart & Neuder, 2001)

According Mahrt, Burfeind & Heuwieser (2014) to measure BHBA, blood samples of continuously fed dairy cows can be drawn at any time of the day. A single measurement provides very good test characteristics for on-farm conditions. Blood samples for BHBA measurement should be drawn from the jugular vein or tail vessels; the mammary vein should not be used for this purpose.

In search for accuracy of milk ketone bodies from flow-injection analysis for the diagnosis of hyperketonemia in dairy cows. Denis-Robichaud, Dubuc, Lefebvre, and DesCôteaux (2014) observed that accounted for milk BHBA and milk acetone values simultaneously had the highest accuracy of all tested models for predicting hyperketonemia. These results support that milk BHBA and milk acetone values from flow-injection analysis are accurate diagnostic tools for hyperketonemia in dairy cows and could potentially be used for herd-level hyperketonemia surveillance programs.

The evaluation of NEFA and BHB represents a strategy for the monitoring of subclinical ketosis and prepartum negative energy balance in dairy cows (Contreras, O'Boyle, Herdt, & Sordillo, 2010). The intravenous Glucose tolerance test (GTT) was useful o studying the physiological adaptation of animals to transition period since it produced a specific insulin response path (Morgante et al., 2012) Treatment should be carried out with the 40% glucose, glucocorticoids, propylene glycol, sodium propionate and B12 (greater propionate production). Should avoid excessive weight loss at calving (management body condition score). The transition of diets should be performed with caution, always carefully to ensure gradual changes in the types of crops, gradual changes in the amounts of concentrates to supply adequate energy levels at different stages of production. Supplementation with niacin (6-12g / d) works best when forages and grains are supplied separately (largest fluctuation of glucose, insulin, NEFA and ketones in the blood) (Wittwer, 2000).

Recent research has demonstrated a reduction in lipoprotein assembly and secretion of TGL can promote deficits choline in non-ruminants. The addition of other methyl donors such as methionine serves to prevent the accumulation of lipids in the liver in mice, perhaps as substrates for the synthesis of choline. Currently there is considerable interest in the use of choline and related compounds to reduce fatty liver associated with the onset of labor. Rumen on the hill is a promise to modulate the metabolism of cows in transition period and reduce the incidence and severity of fatty liver at calving (Figure 4). The frequency response of a significant positive milk production of rumen-protected choline is observed in 50% of studies. Metabolic responses to rumen-protected choline have been mistaken. The predictable response to feeding rumen protected choline may depend on the basal diet, the supply of other B vitamins and related factors, and other management factors, including body condition score of cows entering the transition period (Donkin, 2011). Moreover, the formation of lipoproteins in the liver is not only in dependence of nutrients such as choline but a number of related factors to fat utilization by ruminants that are sensitive to these nutrients because of the deleterious effect that it promotes rumen. Thus, despite advances, little can be said about reducing the incidence of fatty liver by the use of this substance.

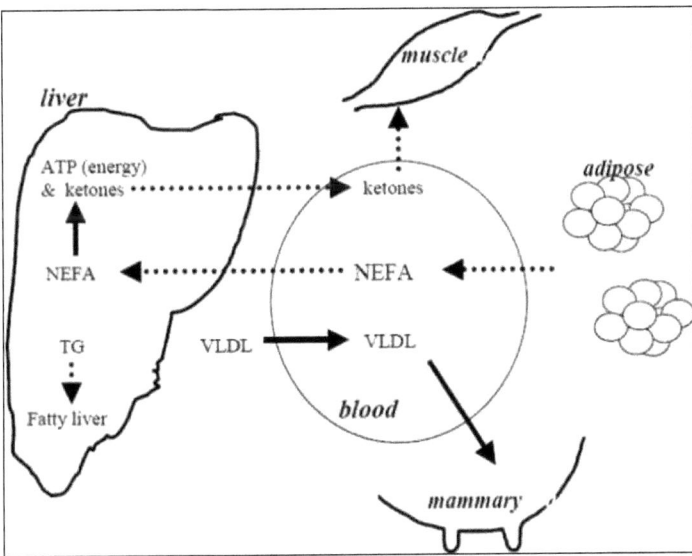

Figure 4. Fat mobilization occurred in cases of fatty liver syndrome or hepatic lipidosis and formation of fat globules in the mammary gland (Grummer, Mashek & Hayirli, 2004)

The prevention is determined that intervention with glucagon as a treatment/prevention of fatty liver is most effective within 14 days after parturition. The results demonstrated that subcutaneous injections of glucagon of 7.5 and 15 mg/d starting at 2 d postpartum are sufficient for fatty liver prevention; however, some cows developed fatty liver already at d 2 postpartum. Previous results confirm (Osman et al., 2008) showing that prenatally and subcutaneously injected glucagon will decrease markedly the accumulation of lipid in the liver of the post parturient dairy cow. Daily administration of the same amount (15 mg/day) of glucagon for several days prenatally in a limited number of cows was effective in preventing fatty liver during the early post parturient period.

## 2.6 Major Metabolic Diseases: Hypocalcemia Dairy Cow or Milk Fever

Hypocalcemia is particularly amenable to strategies tailored to individual cows or targeted groups of cows. First, a substantial proportion of cows are affected by hypocalcemia. The birth and early lactation are periods of too much stress for dairy cows due to the large metabolic challenges that occur in this period (Bezerra et al., 2014). During the last 2 weeks pre-calving, dairy cows are usually in negative energy balance and calcium and, in the last days before calving, the balance of other nutrients such as protein, vitamins and minerals may also be compromised. This reduction in serum calcium concentrations usually occurs about 12 to 24 hours after calving (Figure 4, Kimura, Reinhardt & Goff, 2006; Goff, 2008), where cases of hypocalcemia are more frequent and the most predisposing cows heifers.

Also known as milk fever or puerperal paresis, hypocalcemia is a metabolic-nutritional disease caused by the organism insufficiencies in maintaining serum calcium this period constant transformation in cows. It is a metabolic disease that affects cattle, especially animals with high milk production, which is the lowering of serum calcium and a subsequent number of other problems, such as decubitus and paresis, among others. The etiology is varied but the disease is associated with the delivery and early lactation, causing an exponential increase in needs for calcium (Ca). Calcium is a macromineral that has important functions in the body, among them are the bone matrix, the process of muscle contractor and transmission of nerve impulses. The level of calcium in plasma is well regulated, and when the level decreases, the parathyroid gland will excrete parathyroid hormone (PTH) (Oetzel & Miller, 2012). This increases the mobilization of calcium from the skeleton and also raises the renal threshold for calcium in the kidneys (Goff, Littledike & Horst, 1986). During the dry period, the supply of calcium through the diet is usually more than adequate to maintain homoeostasis without activating the calcium mobilization system (Ramberg, Mayer, Kronfeld, Phang & Berman, 1970), which is thus usually not activated until parturition. It is the phase most important in the development of milk fever (Kronqvist, Ferneborg, Emanuelson & Holtenius, 2014; DeGaris & Lean, 2008).

One of the major complications in the occurrence of hypocalcemia is that as the Ca is responsible for impulses transmission of nerve and muscle contractions, since the problem set and depending on its severity ie the severity of paresis may happen several other secondary disorders of order productive or reproductive due to this muscle inactivity, can cite among others retained placenta, metritis, ruminal acidosis, ketosis, due also to the reduction of dry matter intake and negative energy balance (Goff, 2008; Oetzel, 2011).

The cause is the deficiency of Ca in the early period of lactation. The concentration of plasma calcium is coordinated by action of calciotropic parathyroid hormone (PTH) and 1.25-dihydroxyvitamin D3 [1.25 (OH) 2D3] which are produced in response to hypocalcemia, acting to increase the intake of calcium in the pool plasma. Any decrease in serum calcium stimulates parathyroid gland to secrete PTH which, within minutes, increase renal calcium reabsorption from the glomerular filtrate. If the decreased plasma calcium is small, calcium returns to normal levels and PTH returned to their baseline levels. However, if the calcium drained plasma pool is in large quantities, the continued secretion of PTH stimulates resorption of calcium from bone For a long time it was considered that the tail of the disorder was given due to a failure to respond to release PTH. However, further studies demonstrated that these glands were able to respond to increased demand for calcium, even in cows with puerperal hypocalcemia. Currently it is known that the pathogenesis of the disease is much more associated with the action of PTH on cells responsible for demineralization (osteoclasts), cells of the intestine responsible for absorption and kidney cells responsible for the reabsorption of calcium in the tubules. Factors such as the world Production of milk, age and race are predisposing cows to have the disturbance, since cows for producing more secreted more calcium and should have efficient metabolism to meet increased demand. The great demand of calcium in early lactation to produce 10 liters of colostrum (colostrum formation begins 30 days before calving) cow loses 23 g of calcium in a single milking (2.3 g/L) which is about nine times more present in the plasma compartment. The calcium lost from the plasma compartment should be replaced by intestinal calcium absorbed and bone reabsorption. During the dry season these mechanisms are inactive, and all cows undergo hypocalcemia in the first days after birth until the intestines and bones are adapted. The adaptation starts with increased PTH and 1,25 - (OH) 2D at the beginning of hypocalcemia. About 24 hours of stimulation of 1,25 - (OH) 2D is required for intestinal calcium transport increase significantly. Bone reabsorption (osteoclast recruitment and activation) is not increased until 48 hours after the stimulation of PTH. In cows with parturient paresis this adaptation to these procedures may be extended. In these animals the decline of plasma and extracellular calcium determine the death of the animal before intestinal and bone adaptation (Radostits, Gay, Blood & Hinchcliff, 2002).

Hypocalcemia may or may not show clinical signs. Studies show that many cases of milk fever, animals do not externalize the clinical signs. The most severe hypocalcemia, said clinic (Ca <5 mg / dl), has very serious economic point of view because if not rapidly controlled may lead to loss of the affected animal; On the other hand, subclinical hypocalcemia assumes a more insidious role leading to loss of production and fertility. Subclinical hypocalcemia in which concentrations of calcium in the blood does not decline as severely affects about 50% of lactating dairy cows. If the animals are supplemented with minerals to reduce the risk of milk fever the hypocalcemic percentage of cows is reduced to about 15 to 25% (Oetzel, 2011).

Regarding the clinical signs of the disease in the stage I, the cow is not yet paresis. At this stage of puerperal hypocalcemia, hypersensitivity conductors nerves and muscles occurs, may cause excitement, muscle tremors, anorexia, ataxia, and general debility. The animal does not want to move, do not feed, but often body temperature is normal and may remain in this stage for hours. The stage II is the prodromica phase of the disease and is characterized by prostration and external decumbency. The tetania observed in the first phase is replaced by prolonged external decumbency with the animal unable to stand, displaying paresis, dry muzzle, cold extremities and temperature above normal (36.5 to 38 °C) . The artery pulse is weak, barely audible heart sounds and moderate heart frequency (to 80/min). It is observed absence of ruminal stasis and movements which can lead to a secondary bloat. The stage III is the most advanced, the animal enters and completes lateral decubitus sagging. Cardiac depression is severe and irregular and almost imperceptible pulse, breathing is shallow and diminished. Untreated animals die peacefully with shock in a state of complete collapse (Goff, 1999; Oetzel, 2011).

The diagnosis of milk fever is given based on the history of the animal at birth, age of dam and in the concentrations of calcium in the blood. The decrease in serum levels of magnesium and phosphorus may also be associated. Blood cell count may be some changes as eosinopenia, neutrophilia and lymphopenia suggestive of adrenocortical hyperactivity, but are nonspecific changes. Because of the symptoms is necessary to perform diagnosis differs in relation to hepatic steatosis, septic endometritis, mastitis and acute rumen acidosis. Calcium levels may appear below 5 mg/dl, but with less than 7 mg/dl levels, the animals have demonstrated clinical signs (Figure 5).

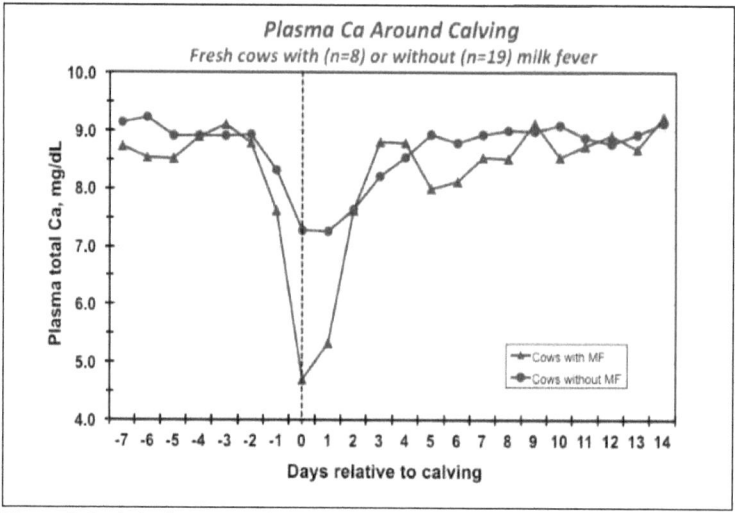

Figure 5. Period of greatest clinical occurrence of milk fever in cows post calving (Adapted Kimura et al. 2006)

The treatment should be carried out as quickly as possible. Animals should be treated as soon as possible. The calcium treated by oral route is the best approach to hypocalcemia cows that are still standing, and the absorption into your bloodstream in about 30 minutes supplementation (Goff & Horst, 1993). The intravenous administration (IV) calcium is not recommended for the treatment of cows that are still standing (Oetzel, 2011), since this application if not done correctly can result in dead animal by cardiac complication. Cows treated with calcium IV often suffer a relapse hypocalcemic 12 to 18 hours later (Curtis, Cote, McLennan, Smart & Rowe, 1978; Thilsing ï

Hansen, Jørgensen, & Østergaard, 2002). For cows in stage II and III of milk fever should be treated immediately with a slow IV administration of 500 ml of a solution of calcium gluconate 23 %. This gives 10.8 g of elemental calcium, which is more than sufficient to correct the deficit whole cow's calcium (about 4 to 6 grams).

Prevention should be performed with the mineral at ease and even forced supplementation during the transition period. In addition to the findings of a larger number of micro minerals essential to functioning of the animal organism, studies have also addressed the relationship between cations and anions present in a certain diet aiding in the metabolic processes of the animal (e.g., acid-base balance) in a particular production phase, thus the anionic and cationic diets have been widely researched and used in animal production, mainly in feeding cows pre - calving, animal class often neglected because the producers are not producing milk and consequently does not contributed directly in net income from property (Oetzel, 2004). One of the main aims of using anionic diets in cows during transition period is control subclinical hypocalcemia, milk fever or puerperal paresis. Hypocalcemia is characterized by rapid depletion of blood calcium levels due to the large demand for calcium to the mammary gland in early lactation. The hormones responsible the absorption of calcium in the intestine so as bones, is low in activity due to small calcium requirement during the dry period. From the moment in which animal has one hypocalcemia, increase the incidence of other metabolic disorders such as mastitis, metritis, uterine prolapsed, retained placenta and ketosis, since calcium is a major responsible for muscle contraction and hence the mineral uterine atony and disposal the placenta.

Sakha, Mahmoudi & Nadalian (2014) in study to determine the effects of varying dietary cation-anion differences (DCAD) in prepartum period on milk fever, subclinical hypocalcemia and negative energy balance in dairy cows showed that use of anionic diets during three weeks before calving can protect dairy cows from clinical and subclinical hypocalcemia by increasing the calcium level in serum. To reduce the postpartum negative energy balance, replacement of anionic diet by cationic ions soon after calving is suggested (Sakha, Mahmoudi, & Nadalian, 2014).

## 3. Conclusions

Metabolic diseases are of great economic impact; it usually affects the animals about to reach their maximum potential production. Food consumption cannot be harmed in the coming days to calving and early lactation, since this is a critical period in the nutrition of females. Is any factor that restricts food intake at this stage (such as milk fever or ketosis) increases the metabolism of body fat, when the animal has in order to obtain energy, with consequent accumulation of fat in the liver immobilized, directly affecting the deficit power of females.

It is accepted that reproduction is important for the profitability of dairy farms, and nutritional status and metabolic health are both associated with successful reproduction. Cows that experience periparturient problems have delayed return to ovulation, lower pregnancy per insemination, and increased pregnancy loss. Therefore, implementing nutritional and health programs that reduce the risk of metabolic disturbances are expected to not only improve cow health, but also enhance fertility. Low nutrient intake coupled with high energy demand during the transition period will increase the risk of occurrence of metabolic disorders. Strategies to manipulate peripartum metabolic health involve dietary formulation to minimize the degree and extent of negative nutrient balance, improve Ca homeostasis, and minimize the severity of negative energy balance.

## 4. Literature Consulted

Andresen, S. H. (2001). Vacas secas y en Transición. *Rev. investig. vet. Perú, 12*(2), 38-46.

Barber, M.C., Clegg, R.A., Travers, M.T., Vernon, R.G. (1997). Lipid metabolism in the lactating mammary gland. *Biochimica et Biophysica Acta,* 1347 101ï 126.

Bauman, D.E. (2000). Regulation of nutrient partitioning during lactation: Homeostasis and homeorhesis revisited. *In:* Ruminant Physiology: Digestion, Metabolism, Growth and Reproduction. CAB;

Bauman, D.E., Currie, W.B. (1980). Partioning of nutrients during pregnancy and lactation: a review of mechanisms involving homeostasis and homeorhesis. *J. Dairy Sci.,* 63: 1514-1529.

Bassett, J. M. (1986). Nutrition of the conceptus: Aspects of its regulation. Proc. Nutr. Soc. 45:l.

Bell, A. W. (1995). Regulation of organic nutrient metabolism during transition from late pregnancy to early lactation. *Journal of Animal Science, 73,* 2804ï 2819.

Bell, A. W. (1993). Pregnancy and fetal metabolism. In: J. M. Forbes and J. France (Ed.) QuantitativeA spects of Ruminant Digestion and Metabolism. p 405. CAB International, Oxford, U . K.

Bell, A. W., M. B. Rymph, R. Slepetis, W. A. House, and R. A. Ehrhardt. (1992). Net nutrient requirements for conceptus growth in Holstein cows - implications for dry cow feeding. *In:* Proc. 1992 Cornell Nutrition Conf. for Feed Manufacturers. p. 102.

Bell, A. W., Bauman, D. E. (1997). Adaptations of Glucose Metabolism During Pregnancy and Lactation. *J Mammary Gland Biol Neoplasia, 2,* 265-278.

Bertics, S. J., Grummer, R. R. (1999). Effects of fat and methionine hydroxy analog on prevention or alleviation of fatty liver induced by feed restriction. *Journal Dairy Science. 82*, 2731ï2736.

Bewley, J. M., Schutz, M. M. (2008). Review: An interdisciplinary review of body condition scoring for dairy cattle. *Prof. Anim. Sci, 24*, 507-529.

Bezerra, L. R., Torreão, J. N. C., Marques, C. A. T., Machado, L. P., Araújo, M. J., & Veiga A. M. S. (2013). Influence of concentrate supplementation and the animal category in the hemogram of Morada Nova sheep. *Arquivo Brasileiro de Medicina Veterinária Zootecnia, 65*(6), 1738-1744.

Bezerra, L. R., Oliveira Neto, C. B., Araújo, M. J., Edvan, R. L., Oliveira, W. D. C., Pereira, F. B. (2014). Major Metabolic Diseases Affecting Cows in Transition Period. *International Journal of Biology*, 6(3): 85-94.

Bobe, G., Young, J. W., Beitz, D. C. (2004). Invited review: Pathology, etiology, prevention, and treatment of fatty liver in dairy cows. *Journal of Dairy Science, 87*, 3105-3124.

Butler, W.R. (2000). Nutritional interactions with reproductive performance in dairy cattle. Anim. Reprod. Sci. 60, 449ï 457. Butler, W.R., 2001. Nutritional effects on resumption of ovarian cyclicity and conception rate in postpartum dairy cows. *Anim. Sci. Occas., 26*: 133ï 145.

Britt, J.H. Follicular develpment and fertility: potential impacts of negative energy balance. In: Proc. National Reproduction Symposiun. Pittsburgh, PA, p. 103-112, 1994.

Kendrick, K.W., Bailey, T.L., Ahmadzdeh, A., et al. (1997). Effects of energy balance on hormonal patterns and recovered oocytes of lactating cows. *J. Dairy Sci.*, v. 80, n.1, p. 151,

Burhans, W. S., Bell, A. W. (1998). *Feeding the transition cow.* Pages 247ï 258 in Proc. Cornell Nutr. Conf. Feed Manuf. Cornell Univ., Ithaca NY.

Burhans, W. S., Bell, A. W., Nadeau, R., Knapp, J. R. (2003). Factors associated with transition cow ketosis incidence in selected New England herds. *Journal Dairy Science*, 86(Suppl. 1):247. (Abstr.)

Butler, W. R. Efeito do balanço energético negativo na fertilidade de vacas leiteiras. In anais do VII curso de novos enfoques na produção e reprodução de bovinos, Uberlândia, 2004.

Chapinal, N., Carson, M. E., LeBlanc, S. J., Leslie, K. E., Godden, S., Capel, M., Duffield, T. F. (2012). The association of serum metabolites in the transition period with milk production and early lactation reproductive performance. *Journal of Dairy Science, 95*, 1301-1309.

Chapinal, N., Carson, M., Duffield, T. F., Capel, M., Godden, S., Overton, M., LeBlanc, S. J. (2011). The association of serum metabolites with clinical disease during the transition period. *Journal of Dairy Science, 94*, 4897-4903.

Chilliard, Y., Remond, B., Sauvant, D., Vermorel, M. (1983). Particularités du métabolisme énergetique. In: Particularités nutritionnelles des vaches à haut potentiel de production. *Bull. Tech. CRZV*, v.53, p.37-64,

Campos, R., González, F., Coldebella, A., Lacerda, L. (2005). Determinação de corpos cetônicos na urina como ferramenta para o diagnóstico rápido de cetose subclínica bovina e relação com a composição do leite. *Archives of Veterinary Science, 10*(2), 49-54.

Canfield, R.W., Sniffen, C.J., Butler, W.R. (1990). Effects of excess degradable protein on post partun reproduction and energy balance in dairy cattle. *J. Dairy Sci.*, v. 73, p. 2342-2349,

Comline, R. S., Silver, M. (1976). Some aspects of foetal and utero-placental metabolism in cows with indwelling umbilical and uterine vascular catheters. *J. Physiol.* (Lond.) 260:57.

Compton, C. W. R., McDougall, S., Young, L., Bryan, M. A. (2014). Prevalence of subclinical ketosis in mainly pasture-grazed dairy cows in New Zealand in early lactation. *New Zealand Veterinary Journal,* 62(1).

Contreras, L. L., Ryan, C. M., Overton, T. R. (2004). Effects of dry cow grouping strategy and prepartum body condition score on performance and health of transition dairy cows. *Journal Dairy Science,* 87: 517ï 523.

Contreras, G. A., O'Boyle, N. J., Herdt, T. H., Sordillo, L. M. (2010). Lipomobilization in periparturient dairy cows influences the composition of plasma nonesterified fatty acids and leukocyte phospholipid fatty acids. *Journal of Dairy Science, 93*: 2508-2516.

Corbett, R. B. (2002). Influence of days fed a close-up dry cow ration and heat stress on subsequent milk production in western dairy herds. *Journal Dairy Science,* 85(Suppl. 1):191ï 192.

Curtis, R. A., Cote, J. F., McLennan, M. C., Smart, J. F., Rowe, R. C. (1978). Relationship of methods of treatment to relapse rate and serum levels of calcium and phosphorous in parturient hypocalcaemia. *Canadian Veterinary Journal, 19*, 155-158.

Curtis, C. R., H. N. Erb, C. H. Sniffen, R. D. Smith, Kronfeld, D. S. (1985). Path analysis of dry period nutrition, postpartum metabolic and reproductive disorders, and mastitis in Holstein cows. *Journal of Dairy Science,* 68, 2347ï 2360.

Dann, H. M., Litherland, N. B., Underwood, J. P., Bionaz, M., Drackley, J. K. (2003). Prepartum nutrient intake has minimal effects on postpartum dry matter intake, serum nonesterified fatty acids, liver lipid and glycogen contents, and milk yield. *Journal Dairy Science,* 86(Suppl. 1):106. (Abstr.)

Dax, E. M., Partilla, J. S., Pineeyro, M. A., Gregerman, R. I. (1990). Altered glucagon- and catecholamine hormone-sensitive adenylyl cyclase responsiveness in rat liver membranes induced by manipulation of dietary fatty acid intake. *Endocrinology* 127, 2236ï 2240.

DeGaris, P. J., Lean, I. J. (2008). Milk fever in dairy cows: A review of pathophysiology and control principles. *Veterinary Journal, 176*, 58-69.

Denis-Robichaud, J., Dubuc, J., Lefebvre, D., DesCôteaux, L. (2014) Accuracy of milk ketone bodies from flow-injection analysis for the diagnosis of hyperketonemia in dairy cows. *Journal of Dairy Science*, http://dx.doi.org/10.3168/jds.2013-6744

Doepel, L., Lapierre, H., Kennelly, J. J. (2002). Peripartum performance and metabolism of dairy cows in response to prepartum energy and protein intake. *Journal Dairy Science, 85*, 2315ï 2334.

Douglas, G. N., Drackley, J. K., Overton, T. R., Bateman, H. G. (1998). Lipid metabolismand production by Holstein cows fed control or high fat diets at restricted or ad libitum intakes during the dry period. *Journal Dairy Science*, 81(Suppl. 1):295. (Abstr.)

Domecq, J. J., Skidmore, A. L., Lloyd, J. W., Kaneene, J. B. (1997). Relationship between body condition scores and milk yield in a large dairy herd of high yielding Holstein cows. *Journal Dairy Science*, 80, 101ï 112.

Donkin, S. S. (2011). Extension Foundation. Americaõs Research-based Learning Network. *Rumen-Protected Cholin*. May 2011. Retrieved 14 april, 2014, from http://www.extension.org:80/pages/26158/ rumen-protected-choline.

Drackley, J. K. (1999). Biology of dairy cows during the transition period: The final frontier? *Journal Dairy Science, 82*, 2259ï 2273.

Ellenberger, H. B., Newlander, J. A., Jones, C. H. (1950). Composition of the bodies of dairy cattle. Bull. Vermont Agric. Exp. Sta. No. 558.

Elphick, M. C., Hull, D., Broughton, F. (1979). The transfer of fatty acids across the sheep placenta. *J. Dev. Physiol.* (Oxf.), 1:31.

Faichney, G. J., White, G. A. (1987). Effects of maternal nutritional status on fetal and placental growth and on fetal urea synthesis in sheep. *Austr. J. Biol. Sci.,* 40:365.

Ferrell, C. L. (1988). Placental regulation of fetal growth. In: D. R. Campion, G. J. Hausman, R. J. Martin (Ed.) *Animal Growth Regulation.*, p.1. Plenum Press, New York.

Ferrell, C. L. (1991). Maternal and fetal influences on uterine and conceptus development in the cow: 11. Blood flow and nutrient flux. *J. Anim. Sci.,* 69:1954.

Ferrell, C. L., W. N. Garrett, and N. Hinman. (1976). Growth, development and composition of the udder and gravid uterus of beef heifers during pregnancy. *J. Anim. Sci.,* 42:1477.

Gillund, P., Reksen O., Grohn Y. T., Karlberg, K. (2001). Body condition related to ketosis and reproductive performance in Norwegian dairy cows. *Journal of Dairy Science, 84*, 1390-1396.

Godden, S. M., Stewart, S. C., Fetrow, J. F., Rapnicki, P., Cady, R., Weiland, W., Spencer, H., Eicker, S. W. (2003). The relationship between herd rbST-supplementation and other factors and risk for removal for cows in Minnesota Holstein dairy herds. Pages 55ï 64 in Proc. Four-State Nutr. Conf. LaCrosse, WI. MidWest Plan Service publication MWPS-4SD16.

Goff, J. P. (1999). Treatment of calcium, phosphorus, and magnesium balance disorders. *Veterinary.*
*Clin. North Am. Food Animal. Pract., 15*, 619-639.

Goff, J. P. (2008). The monitoring, prevention, and treatment of milk fever and subclinical
hypocalcemia in dairy cows. *Veterinary Jour*nal, 176, 50-57.

Goff, J. P., Horst, R. L. (1993). Oral administration of calcium salts for treatment of hypocalcemia in
cattle. *Journal of Dairy Science, 76*, 101-108.

Goff, J. P., Horst, R. L. (1997). Physiological changes at parturition and their relationship to
metabolic disorders. *Journal of Dairy Science, 80*, 1260-1268.

Goff, J. P., Littledike, E. T., Horst, R. L. (1986). Effect of synthetic bovine parathyroid hormone in
dairy cows: prevention of hypocalcemic parturient paresis. *Journal of Dairy Science, 69*,
2278-2289.

Garnsworthy,P. C., Topps, J.H. (1982a). The effect of body condition of dairy cows at calving on
their food intake and performance when given complete diets. *Anim. Prod. 35*,113ï 119.

Garnsworthy, P. C., Topps, J. H. (1982b). The effects of body condition at calving, food intake, and
performance in early lactation on blood composition of dairy cows given complete diets. *Anim.*
*Prod. 35*, 121ï 125.

Garnsworthy, P. C., Jones, G. P. (1987). The influence of body condition at calving and dietary
protein supply on voluntary food intake and performance in dairy cows. *Anim. Prod. 44*,
347ï 353.

Grant, R.J., Albright, D.J. (1995). Feeding behavior and management factors during the transition
period in dairy cattle. *J. Anim. Sci.*, v. 73, p. 2791.

Gross, J. J., Schwarz, F. J., Eder, K., Van Dorland, H. A., Bruckmaier, R. M. (2013). Liver fat content and lipid metabolism in dairy cows during early lactation and during a mid-lactation feed restriction. *Journal of Dairy Science, 96*, 5008-5017. http://dx.doi.org/10.3168/jds.2012-6245.

Grum, D. E., Drackley, J. K., Younker, R. S., LaCount, D. W., Veenhuizen, J. J. (1996). Nutrition during the dry period and hepatic lipid metabolism of periparturient dairy cows. *Journal Dairy Science, 79*, 1850ï1864.

Grummer, R. R., Carroll, D. J. (1991). Effects of dietary fat on metabolic disorders and reproductive performance of dairy cattle. *Journal of Animal Science. 69*, 3838ï3852.

Grummer, R. R. (1993). Etiology of lipid-related metabolic disorders in periparturient dairy cows. Journal Dairy Science, *76,* 3882ï3896.

Grummer, R. R. (1995). Impact of changes in organic nutrient metabolism on feeding the transition dairy cow. *Journal of Animal Science, 73*, 2820ï2833.

Grummer, R. R., Mashek, D. G., Hayirli, A. (2004). Dry matter intake and energy balance in the transition period. *Vet Clin North Am Food, Anim Pract, 20*, 447-470.

Guesnet, P. M., Massoud, M. J., Demarne, Y. (1991). Regulation of adipose tissue metabolism during pregnancy and lactation in the ewe: the role of insulin. *Journal Animal Science, 69*, 2057-2065.

Hammon, D.S., Evjen, I.M., Dhiman, T.R., Goff, J.P., Walters, J.L. (2006). Neutrophil function and energy status in Holstein cows with uterine health disorders. *Ve Immunol Immunopath, 113,* 21ï29.

Hay, W. W., Myers, S. A., Sparks J. W., Wilkening, R. B., Meschia, G., Battaglia, F. C. (1983). Glucose and lactate oxidation rates in the fetal lamb. *Proc. Soc. Exp. Biol. Med.* 173:553.

Hayirli, A., Grummer, R. R., Nordheim, E. V., Crump, P. M. (2002). Animal and dietary factors affecting feed intake during the prefresh transition period in Holsteins. *Journal Dairy Science.* *85*, 3430ï 3443.

Heidrich, H.D., Gruner, J., Vaske,T. R. (1980) *Enfermidades Metabólicas e Carências. Manual de Patologia Bovina*, J. M Varela livros LTDA. São Paulo, pp. 191-192,

Herdt, T. H., Dart, B., Neuder, L. (2001). Will large dairy herds lead to the revival of metabolic profile testing? *Proc Am Assoc Bov Pract, 34*, 27-34.

Holtenius, P. (1991). Disturbances in the regulation of energy metabolism around parturition in cows. *Mh. Vet.-Med, 46*, 795-797.

Kehrli M.E., Nonecke B.J., Roth J.A. (1989). Alterations in bovine neutrophil function during the periparturient period. *Am J Vet Res, 50*, 207ï 214.

Kimura, K., Goff J.P., Kehrli, M.E., Reinhardt, T.A. (2002). Decreased neutrophil function as a cause of retained placenta in dairy cattle. *Journal Dairy Science, 85,* 544ï 550.

Kimura, K., Reinhardt, T. A., Goff, J. P. (2006). Parturition and hypocalcemia blunts calcium signals in immune cells of dairy cattle. *Journal of Dairy Science, 89*, 2588-2595.

Kumamoto, T., Ide, T. (1998). Comparative effects of $\check{U}$ and Ɔ-linolenic acids on rat liver fatty acid oxidation. *Lipids* 33, 647ï 654.

Kronqvist, C., Ferneborg, S., Emanuelson, U., Holtenius, K. (2014). Effects of pre-partum milking of dairy cows on calcium metabolism at start of milking and at calving. *Journal of Animal Physiology and Animal Nutrition, 98*(1), 191-196.

Kronfeld, D. S. (1982). Major metabolic determinants of milk volume, mammary efficiency, and spontaneous ketosis in dairy cows. *Journal Dairy Science.* 65, 2204ï 2212.

Lambert, M. S., Avella, M. A., Botham, K. M., Mayes, P. A. (1998). Comparison of short- and long-term effects of different dietary fats on hepatic uptake and metabolism of chylomicron remnants in rats. *Br. J. Nutr.* 79, 203ï 211.

Lemons, J. A., Adcock, E. W., Jones Jr. , M. D., Naughton, M. A., Meschia, G., Battaglia, F. C. (1976). Umbilical uptake of amino acids in the unstressed fetal lamb. *J. Clin. Invest.* 58: 1428.

Leroy, J. L. M. R., Vanholder, T., Van Knegsel, A.T. M., Garcia-Ispierto, I., Bols, P. E. J. (2008). Nutrient Prioritization in Dairy Cows Early Postpartum: Mismatch Between Metabolism and Fertility? *Reprod Domest Anim, 43*(Suppl.), 96-103.

Lucy M. (2004). Mechanisms linking the somatotropic axis with insulin: Lessons from the postpartum dairy cow. *Proc NZ Soc Anim Prod*, 64, 19ï 23.

Lucy, M. C., Crooker, B. A. (2001). Physiological and genetic differences between low and high index dairy cows. In: Fertility in the High Producing Dairy Cow. *British Society of Animal Science Occas.* 26:223ï 236.

Mahrt, A., Burfeind, O., Heuwieser, W. (2014). Effects of time and sampling location on concentrations of β-hydroxybutyric acid in dairy cows. *Journal of Dairy Science, 97*(1), 291-298.

Mallard, B. A., Dekkers, J. C., Ireland, M. J., Leslie, K. E., Sharif, S., Lacey Vankampen, C., Wagter, L., Wilkie, B. N. (1998). Alteration in immune responsiveness during the peripartum period and its ramification on dairy cow and calf health. *Journal Dairy Science, 81,* 585ï 595.

Malewiak, M. I., Rozen, R., Le Liepvre, X., Griglio, S. (1988). Oleate metabolism and endogenous triacylglycerol hydrolysis in isolated hepatocytes from rats fed a high-fat diet. *Diabetes Metab.*, 14, 270ï 276.

Mashek, D. G., Beede, D. K. (2001). Peripartum responses of dairy cows fed energy-dense diets for 3 or 6 weeks prepartum. *J. Dairy Sci.*, 84:115ï 125.

Martinez, N., Sinedino, L. D. P., Bisinotto, R. S., Ribeiro, E. S., Gomes, G. C., Lima, F. S., Santos J. E. P. (2014). Effect of induced subclinical hypocalcemia on physiological responses and neutrophil function in dairy cows. *Journal of Dairy Science,* 97(2), 874ï 887.

Matos, L.L. (1995). Perspectivas em alimentação e manejo de vacas em lactação. *In:* Anais da XXXII Reunião Anual da SBZ. Anais, Brasília ï DF, 1995, p.147-155.

Meier, P. R., Teng, C., Battaglia, F. C., Meschia, G. (1981). The rate of amino acid nitrogen and total nitrogen accumulation in the fetal lamb. *Proc. Soc. Exp. Biol. Med.,* 167:463.

Meier, P. R., Teng, C., Battaglia, F. C., Meschia, G. (1981). The rate of amino acid nitrogen and total nitrogen accumulation in the fetal lamb. *Proc. Soc. Exp. Biol. Med.,* 167:463.

Meschia, G., Battaglia, F. C., Hay Jr., W. W., Sparks, J. W. (1980). Utilization of substrates by the ovine placenta in vivo. *Fed. Proc.,* 39:245.

Meznarich, H. K., Hay Jr., W. W., Sparks, J. W., Meschia, G., Battaglia, F. C. (1987). Fructose disposal and oxidation rates in the ovine fetus. *Q. J. Exp. Physiol.,* 72:617.

Morgante, M., Gianesella, M., Casella, S., Stelletta, C., Cannizzo, C., Giudice, E., Piccione, G. (2012). Response to glucose infusion in pregnant and nonpregnant ewes: changes in plasma glucose and insulin concentrations. *Comp Clin Pathol, 21*, 961-965.

National Animal Health Monitoring System. (2008). Dairy 2007 Part I: Reference of Dairy Cattle Health and Management Practices in the United States, 2007. USDA

Nutrient Requirements of Dairy Cattle - NRC. (1988). (6th Rev. Ed.). National Academy Press, Washington, DC.

Nutrient Requirements of Dairy Cattle - NRC. (1989). Nutrient requeriments of dairy cattle. Sixth Revised Edition, 157 p.

National Research Council. (2001). *Nutrient Requirements of Dairy Cattle.* 7th rev. ed.

National Research Council. (2007). *Nutrient Requirements of Dairy Cattle.* 8th rev. ed.

Nielsen, N. I., Ingvartsen, K. L. (2004). Propylene glycol for dairy cows: A review of the metabolism of propylene glycol and its effects on physiological parameters, feed intake, milk production and risk of ketosis. *Anim Feed Sci Technol,* 115, 191-213.

Oetzel, G. R. (2004). Monitoring and testing dairy herds for metabolic disease. *Veterinary Clin. North Am. Food Animal. Pract, 20,* 651-674.

Oetzel, G. R. (2011). Non-infectious diseases: Milk fever. *In* J. W. Fuquay & P. L. H. McSweeney (Eds.), *Encyclopedia of Dairy Sciences* (Vol. 2, pp. 239-245). San Diego: Academic Press.

Oetzel, G. R., Miller, B. E. (2012). Effect of oral calcium bolus supplementation on early lactation health and milk yield in commercial dairy herds. *Journal of Dairy Science,* 95, 7051-7065.

Olson, J. (2002). *Estratégias de nutrición para vacas en transición.* Hoard's Dairyman, no. 88, abril, p. 288,

Osman, M. A., Allen, P. S., Mehyar, N. A., Bobe, G., Coetzee, J. F., Koehler, K. J., Beitz, D. C. (2008). Acute metabolic responses of postpartal dairy cows to subcutaneous glucagon injections, oral glucagon, or both. *Journal of Dairy Science,* 91, 3311-3322.

Overton, T. R., Waldron, M. R. (2004). Nutritional Management of Transition Dairy Cows: Strategies to Optimize Metabolic Health. *J. Dairy Sci.,* 87, 105ï 119.

Palmquist, D. L. (1994). The role of dietary fats in efficiency of ruminants. *J. Nutr., 124*, 1377ï 1382.

Pickket, M.M., Piepenbrik, M.S., Overton, T.R. (2003). Effects of propylene glycol or fat drench on plasma metabolites, liver composition, and production of dairy cows during the periparturient period. *Journal of Dairy Science,* 86 : 6.

Piccione, G., Messina, V., Marafioti, S., Casella, S., Giannetto, C., Fazio, F. (2012). Changes of some haematochemical parameters in dairy cows during late gestation, post partum, lactation and dry periods. *Vet Med Zoot, 58*, 59-64.

Radostits, O. M., Gay, C. C., Blood, D. C., Hinchcliff, K. W. (2002). *Clínica veterinária. Um tratado de doenças dos bovinos, ovinos, suínos, caprinos e eqüinos* (Vol. 9, pp. 1737). Rio de Janeiro: Guanabara Koogan.

Ramberg, C. F., Mayer, G. P., Kronfeld, D. S., Phang, J. M., Berman, M. (1970) Calcium kinetics in cows during late pregnancy, parturition, and early lactation. *The American Journal of Physiology, 219*, 1166-1177.

Reynolds, L. P., Ferrell, C. L., Robertson, D. A., Ford, S. P. (1986). Metabolism of the gravid uterus, foetus and utero-placenta at several stages of gestation in cows. *J. Agric. Sci.,* 106:437.

Santos, G.T., Prado, I.N., Branco, A.F. *Aspectos do manejo do gado leiteiro especializado.* Universidade Estadual de Maringá. 1993. 23 p. (Apontamentos, 22).

Santos, J.E.P. *Effect of degree of fatness prepartum on lactational performance and follicular development of early lactation dairy cows.* M.Sc. Thesis. Dept. Animal Scicence, University of Arizona, Tucson, AZ, 1996.

Santos, J.E.P., Thatcher, W.W., Chebel, R.C., Cerri, R.L.A., Galvão, K.N. (2004). The effect of embryonic death rates in cattle on the efficacy of estrous synchronization programs. *Anim. Reprod. Sci.,* 82-83:513-535.

Santos, J. E. P. Efeitos da nutrição e do manejo periparto na eficiência reprodutiva de vacas de leite. *In:* Anais do VIII curso de novos enfoques na produção e reprodução de bovinos. Uberlândia, 2005.

Santos, J. E. P., Sá Filho, M.F. *Biotecnologia da reprodução em bovinos.* 2° Simpósio Internacional de Reprodução Animal Aplicada. São Paulo. 2006.

Skaar, T. C., Grummer, R. R., Dentine, M. R., Stauffacher, R. H. (1989). Seasonal effects of prepartum and postpartumfat and niacin feeding on lactation performance and lipid metabolism. *J. Dairy Sci.,* 72:2028ï2038.

Smith, K. L., Todhunter, D. A., Schoenberger, P. S. (1985). Environmental mastitis: cause, prevalence, prevention. *J. Dairy Sci.,* 68:1531ï1553.

Sakha, M., Ameri, M., Rohbakhsh, A. (2006). Changes in blood ß-hydroxybutyrate and glucose concentrations during dry and lactation periods in Iranian Holstein cows. *Comp Clin Pathol, 15,* 221-226.

Sakha, M., Mahmoudi, M., Nadalian, M. G. (2014). Effects of dietary cation-anion difference on milk fever, subclinical hypocalcemia and negative energy balance in transition dairy cows. *Journal Research Opinions in Animal and Veterinary Sciences, 4*(2), 69-73.

Sasaki, S. (2002). Mechanism of insulin action on glucose metabolism in ruminants. *Anim Sci J, 73*, 423-433.

Seal, C. J., Reynolds, C. K. (1993). Nutritional implications of gastrointestinal and liver metabolism in ruminants. *Nutr. Res. Rev., 6*,185ï 208.

Scalia D., Lacetera N., Bernabucci U. (2006). In vitro effects of nonesterified fatty acids on bovine neutrophils oxidative burst and viability. *Journa Dairy Science,* 89: 147ï 154.

Sheldon, I.M., Lewis, G.S., LeBlanc, S., Gilbert, R. (2006) Defining post partum uterine disease in cattle. *Theriogenology* 65:1516ï 1530.

Sordillo, L.M., Aitken, S.L. (2009). Impact of oxidative stress on the health and immune function of dairy cattle. *Vet Immunol Immunopath,* 128: 104ï 109.

Souza, R. C. (2003). *Considerações sobre desordens metabólicas em vacas leiteiras.* Clinica de Ruminante ï Universidade Federal de Minas Gerais,

Sun, L. W., Zhang, H. Y., Wu, L., Shu, S., Xia, C., Xu, C., & Zheng, J.S. (2014). H-Nuclear magnetic resonance-based plasma metabolic profiling of dairy cows with clinical and subclinical ketosis. *Journal of Dairy Science, 97*(3), 1552-1562.

Thilsing-Hansen, T., Jørgensen R. J., Østergaard, S. (2002). Milk fever control principles: areview. *Acta. Vet. Scand, 43*, 1-19.

Treacher, R. J., Reid, I. M., Roberts, C. J. (1986). Effect of body condition at calving on the health and performance of dairy cows. *Anim. Prod.,* 43:1ї6.

Thacher, W. W. (2005). Dinâmica no período periparto e subseqüente impacto na fertilidade. *In*: Anais do VIII curso de novos enfoques na produção e reprodução de bovinos. Uberlândia.

Vernon, R. G. (1981). Lipid metabolism in the adipose tissue of ruminant animals. *In:* W. W. Christie (Ed.) Lipid Metabolism in Ruminant Animals. p 279. Pergamon Press, Oxford, U. K.

Vernon, R.G., Pond, C.M. (1997). Adaptations of maternal adipose tissue to lactation. *Journal of Mammary Gland Biology and Neoplasia,* 2231ї241.

Villa-Godoy, A., Hughes, T.L., Emery, R.S., Chapin, C.T., Fogwell, R.L. (1988). Association between energy balance and luteal function in lactating dairy cows. *Journal of Dairy Science,* Champaign, 71(4): 1063-1072.

Wathes D.C., Fenwick, M., Cheng Z., Bourne, N., Llewellyn, S., Morris, D.G., Kenny, D., Murphy J., Fitzpatrick, R. (2007). Influence of negative energy balance on cyclicity and fertility in the high producing dairy cow. *Theriogenology* , 68, S232ї S241.

Wathes, D. C., Cheng, Z., Chowdhury, W., Fenwick, M. A., Fitzpatrick, R., Morris, D. G., Murphy, J. J. (2009). Negative energy balance alters global gene expression and immune responses in the uterus of postpartum dairy cows. *Physiol Genomics, 39*, 1-13.

Wittwer, F. (2000). Diagnóstico dos desequilíbrios metabólicos de energia em rebanhos bovinos. In F. H. D. González, J. O. Barcellos, H. Ospina, & L. A. O. Ribeiro (Eds.), *Perfil metabólico em ruminantes: seu uso em nutrição e doenças nuricionais.* Porto Alegre, Brasil, Gráfica da Universidade Federal do Rio Grande do Sul.

Yang, E. K., Radominska, A., Winder, B. S. Dannenberg, A. J. (1993). Dietary lipids coinduce xenobiotic metabolizing enzymes in rat liver. *Biochim. Biophys. Acta, 1168*, 52ï 58.

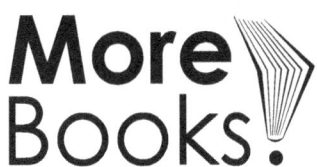
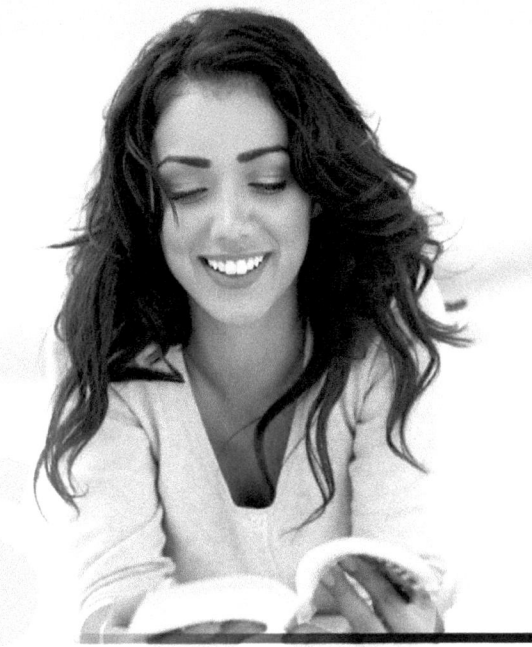

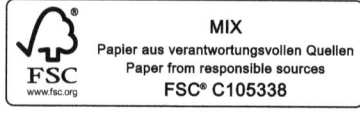

Printed by Books on Demand GmbH, Norderstedt / Germany